NINJA CURE:
The Essence of Health

NINJA CURE:
The Essence of Health

yasuhirA iDee

2014

First Printing: 2014

ISBN 978-1-312-01644-6

<TAIONDOU CLINIC>
201 Hamami Schloss
1-15-5 Tsujido Higashikaigan
Fujisawa, Kanagawa
251-0045 Japan

https://www.facebook.com/yasuhira.ide

http://instagram.com/yasuhira_idee

http://www.oqjin.com

Dedication

To my life partner, friends, mentor and patients.
Thank you. Without your support and patience,
I would have never achieved my dream.

Contents

Acknowledgements

I would like to thank here all the people that have supported yasuhirA iDee in the long run. Our sincerest thanks to all of them!

More particularly we would like to here to thank:

Kenshi Nabeshima / Acupuncture

Mariko Hashimoto / Acupuncture

Dr. Masaaki Matsubara

Donald Gagner / Proof-reading

"Everything that exists around the world is a teacher." The words that I learned from my mentor always remind me of the importance of a grateful feeling for each event. What I inherited from them has evolved by my daily effort and research. Genuinely, thanks for the opportunity to share the achievements with everyone in the world. I hope you, each and every one who has a soul all over the world, have a happy, healthy life :) Thanks.

Preface

Life is art. I believe this tip. Well, there are no people that do not desire to make their dreams come true. That's life, isn't it? I'd love to use this word "art" as a positive verb, including creatively, healthy and comfortably means. Moreover, many people may regard art stuff as only for people with special talents. I say there is no such thing. Art never chooses people. You can do art anytime, and even try any number of times. I say that only two words can change your life to happiness: "Balance" and "Temperature". There's no doubt that it's necessary for art's sense of balance. Temperature means passion in your body and soul. So, art is a big tip for your success.

In my opinion, wellness and art come from same place creative. Always, passion and a well-thinking brain would be fine. Passion and knowledge are necessities for your dream coming true. Both of them are the cure for your trouble, as well. How to resolve, when you're in trouble? How to have a vision of happiness for your bright future? So, I want you to spend your life as a wonderful artist who creates healthy "every days" from right now. As a matter of fact, you already have what you need to have an art life. All right everyone, I as am known as "Ninja", yasuhirA iDee is going to instruct you in how to boost/progress what you need as you read on.

Introduction

Do you like movies? I do. For example, please imagine that you are the artist of your own life. You are a stunning movie star named "Your Life". Your life deserves happiness full of beautiful smiles. So, your smiles are great pieces in "Your Life". That is to say, "smiles live in details, whatever you're going to be". Moreover, here are famous words: "All the world's a stage, and all the men and women are merely players," from William Shakespeare's "As You Like It". Please allow me to add these words: I'd like to change "merely players" to "amazing performers", because, again, you have all you need to play on the stage/life originally. To sum up, the point is how to boost yourself for your happy, healthy life.

I believe your entire life, each piece, is amazingly original. According to recent research of science, the brain gets an illusion. The power of imagination. I believe that the world must become peaceful when healthy people are increased more. Actually, it doesn't matter what your age, gender, race, occupation, diagnosis, etc is. Here is a tip: smiles play an important role in your healthy progress.

Smile is a joy.
Smile is a vibration.
Smile is a virus.
Smile is an infection.
Smile is a cure.
Smile is a hero.
Smile is a family.
Smile is a friend.
Smile is a mentor.
Smile is an idol.
Smile, Smile, Smile :)

Wellness loves smiles.

Nothing beats smiles :D

I hope that a lot of smiles flourish all over the world :)
Therefore, I'm taking my selfie-photos every morning,
hilariously. If you don't mind, please check my
Instagram @yasuhirA_iDee out :) So, I put some of
those selfies and my art shots in this book. I hope you
enjoy them, as well.

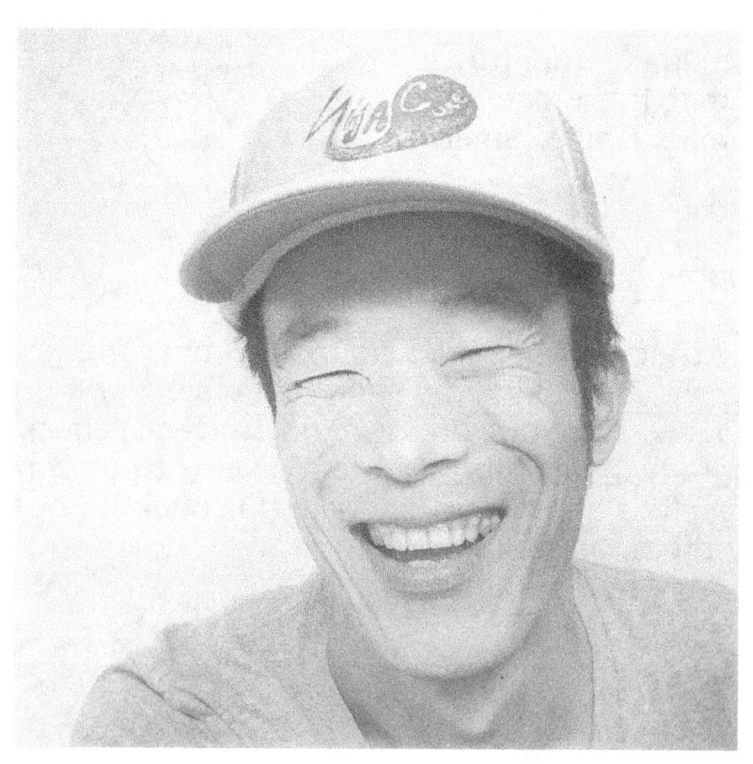

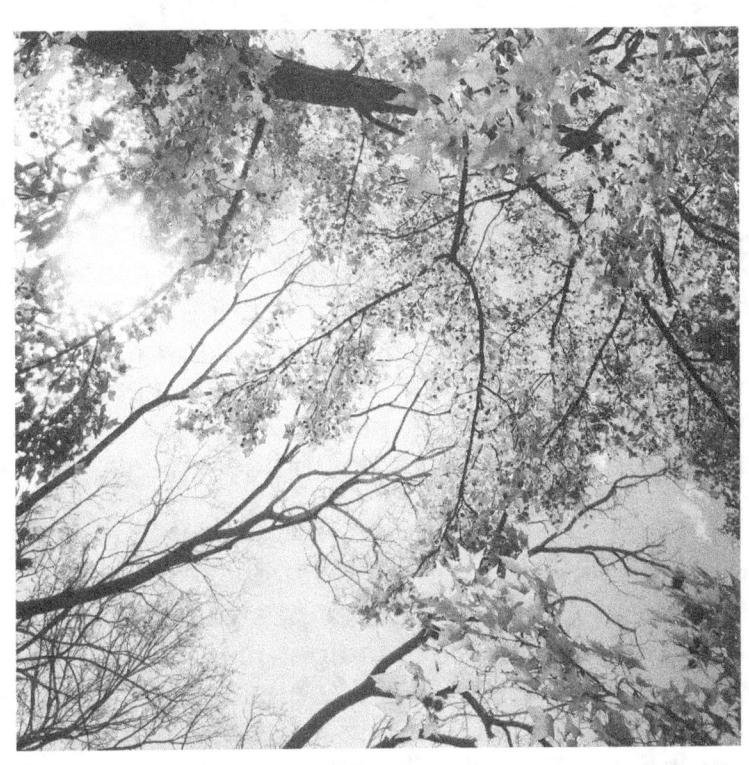

Chapter 1: Boost Wealth/Talent

You know that there is a point of view that some are winners and some are losers in life. Why is that? Just because winners have the talent? I don't think so. No winners without everyday effort. Winners show off amazing performances daily. So, which group will you join? Even if you are a winner, you might not satisfy your achievement goal. Have you ever thought that you do not have any talent, or that you deserved a quality of life more than present? Do you know that you can rediscover/boost a talent with health? Yes, health literally. As previously stated, you already have what you need for art/healthy life. Now, here is a tip for your success story from now on. The essence of health- *Ninja Cure*: I offer you a genuine, successful and safe method that was really organized by my knowledge and experiences of many years. It has already helped a lot of people- my wife, family, friends and my everyday patients, including myself.

It is said that nobody makes money without health. In terms of expense, actually, *Ninja Cure* doesn't cost much money. One tip- the recipes that I introduce in this book are made of vegetables you can get anywhere in the world. To be honest with you, you'll be rich with continuous efforts, because you will have become healthy, gradually while saving money.

In short, *Ninja Cure* is money. There are no following articles containing content that sells any kind of products like fitness tools or supplements. But, I provide you with tips and answers to all of them, including weight-loss, cleansing, relief and boost. Again, the wonderful remedy *Ninja Cure* is a totally genuine, successful, safe and less expensive method.

Recently, "WaShoku" or "Mottainai" are in the spotlight as healthy, even peaceful thoughts all over the world. As you may know, the healthy Food-Cure Recipe can boost/cleanse even each of the cells in your body. Thoughts of *Ninja Cure* based on the Japanese culture can be a tip to lead you to a successful life full of your beautiful smiles. Finally, you're going to get wellness into your happy life.

As a matter of fact, I used to have weakness and was in danger of my health. But fortunately, I'm now healthy, thanks to kind key persons and great remedies. That's why I provide the Idea about *Ninja Cure,* as a survivor from my sickly days. I genuinely want to share the useful idea *Ninja Cure* with many people who need it. I hope you'll enjoy it I provide/produce:) Thanks:)

Chapter 2: The Relief

I am healthy: To begin with, there is no doubt whatever about that. Moreover, I live as well as an artist.

To be honest with you, I believe, from my own knowledge and experiences, "Health/Beauty is an art, won by 99%-SelfCare and 1%-genuine treatment." I might be inclined, to regard art as the most beautiful piece of our life. But the wisdom of our ancestors might have a different opinion. Please, therefore, permit me to repeat, emphatically, that I live as well as an artist.

Ninja knows I am healthy? Of course Ninja does. How could it be otherwise? Ninja and I have been partners for many years. Ninja is my doctor, mentor, family, friend and hero, definitely. The memories of my medical history, especially a hip-joint's operation, brings me back to the point where I started.

My left leg is shorter by an inch compared with my right leg. The cause was a natural born condition. I have always walked with a limp, had the experience of being picked on. There were various issues with my unbalanced body, such as: chronic pains in the neck, shoulder and hip-waist. In my childhood, I tended to have fevers and had a tonsillectomy and pulmonary tuberculosis.

Limitation has come, literally. And then, I had surgery of the hip joint at the age of 30. I've survived to live somehow from the surgery, bleeding 2 liters, and my fever fluctuated up and down around 39 degrees for three weeks. After the hospital discharge, and rehabilitation of a long term, I have still spent entire days with regular pain and fever once a month, at least. No artificial medication has helped my problems. Of course my hip joint is balanced better than before. I believe the doctor also did his best. Thanks to all of them.

Having said that, I still had problems of my body. I have come to try many treatments except Western Medicine: Foods, Reflexology, Seitai; including alternative medicine, natural remedies, etc. In the meantime, I has even qualified as an acupuncturist, including moxa. At that time, there was a little bright sign with my problems. I began to realize the magnificence and effectiveness of the natural remedies. I am genuinely grateful for amazing encounters with great teachers; I really mean it. Those wonderful encounters meant a lot for my revival. Especially, Ninja meant a lot to me. As a matter of fact, one of those reliefs, I had been getting my feet badly frost-bitten every winter since I was a child. But it has no longer happened since the winter of 2009. Not only pains of my inner body, but also other the symptoms, were relieved progressively. There it is. The state of my entire body has totally turned into a wellness direction, feeling cozy. I feel exactly like I have been reborn.

So, what Ninja is all about? You may think, well, that sounds like training of samurai? A master of swordplay? No, but not bad ideas? Haha! You know what? Here, Ninja means a method for health and beauty, and revolutionary fresh vegetable stuff, as well. The Essence of Health results from *Ninja Cure*. All of them are based on true stories and thoughts of those who have gone before. Achievements of myself, my wife, family, friends and my patients. Those things have progressed to more successful remedies that have been organized well during my treatments and my life.

The following article contains content that has expression full of wisdom in Japanese-style. So, imaginative discretion is advised, please read carefully. I think it's very important to write with my own words and is necessary to, as well. I want to tell my successful experiences and achievable thoughts to you more realistically. I hope you become healthy and happy by learning a lot with smile. Thank you:) Good luck:)

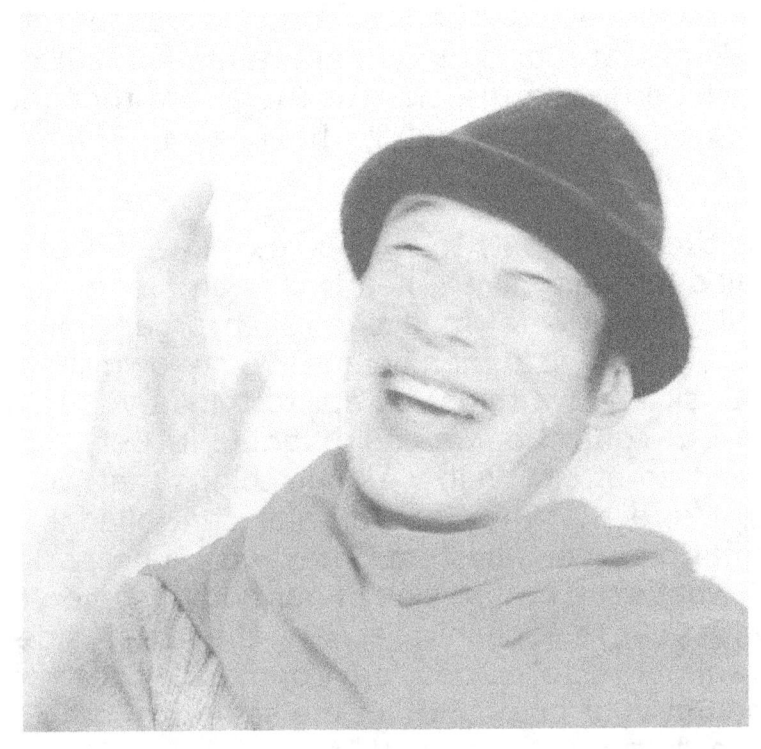

Chapter 3: Wa-Shoku

In 2013, UNESCO, the U.N. cultural organization, added traditional Japanese cuisine, or "Wa-Shoku," into its Intangible Cultural Heritage list. "Wa" means Japanese or Harmony, "Shoku" means to-eat or meal or anything food-related. For Japanese, food is associated with many things. First of all, it means harmony for each one of us; In other words, nutrition's ingredients are also very important; and also the appreciation of nature. That comes from thoughts of shinto: all things in nature have soul. Shinto has existed for over 2,600 years.

Those thoughts apply to our bodies, as well. Our body contains organs: liver, heart, spleen, lung, kidney typically. In oriental medicine, each organ has soul. You know that we human beings live our own life every day. Basically, we might be apt to think everything is under our control or we could handle it. But, actually we can't so often. Well, we have things that we can't control directly. They are organs controlled by the automatic nervous system. They work unconsciously 24/7. That's the nature side of our body. Is everything OK with your relationship between the nature side and the animal side? Does environmental destruction happen in your body? So, let me say again that: Only two words can change your life:

Balance,　Temperature

It is generally said that our immune functions drop down by 30-40% when we decrease our body temperature by 1 degree. We can balance well by ourselves, originally. The issues of balance and temperature cause most chronic diseases and many troubles of your body and mind. As you know, the human body works successfully when the blood spreads evenly in every part of the whole body: Of course, the brain, heart and sensory organs, like the ear and eye, hypothalamus, etc. The hypothalamus is the playmaker of the autonomic nervous system, that plays a crucial role in the function of our nature side; literally, in every organ you have. Moreover, they are all made of cells. The activation of cells requires oxygen and moderate nutrition. What brings the nutrients and oxygen? Yes, your blood.

Have you ever heard of the Japanese, "Mottainai". Wangari Maathai, who was awarded the 2004 Nobel Peace Prize, had used as her motto, "Mottainai". This Japanese term means "a sense of regret concerning waste when the intrinsic value of an object or resource is not properly utilized; and a sense of positive thoughts about appreciation and respect for all things in nature, as well." It is also common to the concept of "Wa-Shoku" in the sense that it respects the personality of the materials themselves.

To sum up: there is no reason not to utilize natural healing power first. Even if you are in a serious situation, you could add *Ninja Cure* to your daily routine. Of course, in that case, it's important that you ask the opinion of your own health-care professional. You know that Western Medicine is mainstream now. I think that's great, but Oriental Medicine is still important/useful for our daily health, especially. Please cure naturally first, as much as possible. Let your natural healing power go well. Certainly, both medicines have a strong field for each other. For instances, such as infectious disease, emergency medical treatment and surgical technique, Western Medicine has been developed and studied in those fields, particularly. But chronic diseases, such as lifestyle-related diseases, have kept increasing. Those have been explained by data of the WHO. Improving the lifestyle is obviously a strong field of Oriental Medicine, as a natural cure.

Remember:

"Health/Beauty is an art, won by 99%-SelfCare and 1%-genuine treatment."

You might have tried a number of ways to become/keep healthy already. Have they worked? You're not good enough? Never give up on your health and beauty. As previously stated, they will all result in your success, wealth and wellness. Why don't you share these wonderful thoughts of *Ninja Cure* and make dreams come true? *Ninja Cure* helps you and makes you smile beautifully. I mean it! So, let's get started!

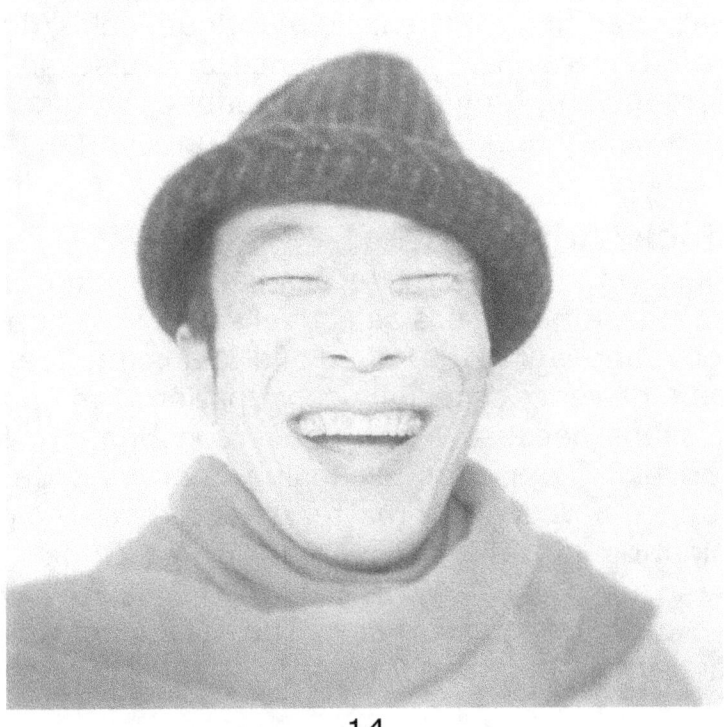

Chapter 4: 3 Steps of "Ninja Cure"

The 3 Revolutionary steps to add *Ninja Cure* into your routine/life daily!

1. Have Ninja Salad/Drink 5 days per week.
2. Eat Black/Adzuki Bean 5 days per week.
3. Smilefie every morning.

Description:

1. Ninja Salad/Drink

I usually have *Ninja Drink* in the morning, and *Ninja Salad* in the evening. I've been drinking it every day since October, 2009. Don't eat hastily, without proper chewing, and you should chew at least 32 times per one bite, because the motion of chewing promotes the secretion of saliva. You can prevent overeating when you eat salad first, in the case of fatigue, colds/flu and before/after training, performance and disease. You can arrange the timing and the quantity to take, and also add honey or agave nectar to it until you get used to its taste.

2. Black/Adzuki Bean

The best way to take these beans is with their soup. Both of these beans are selectively used: black beans for boost and warmth, and adzuki beans for cleansing and as a diuretic, especially constipation. I mainly eat black beans because I don't have constipation, but I eat adzuki beans for cleansing/improving fatigue about once a week. As a matter of fact, there is a great combination between *Ninja Salad/Drink* and Black/Adzuki Beans. *Ninja Salad/Drink* is raw, while Black/Adzuki Beans are warm. The balance of raw and warm stuff should keep you well.

3. Smilefie

Smilefie is made of a smile and a selfie, which means hilariously taking a picture of yourself with your beautiful smile. Remember, wellness loves smiles, and your face stands for your states of health. Moreover, by uploading on Instagram or Facebook, like any other sns, you can have a good sense of tension. I believe that causes the motivation to say, "I deserve wellness, I can do it!" Now, let's get started with *smilefie,* based on refreshing motivation. More information below:

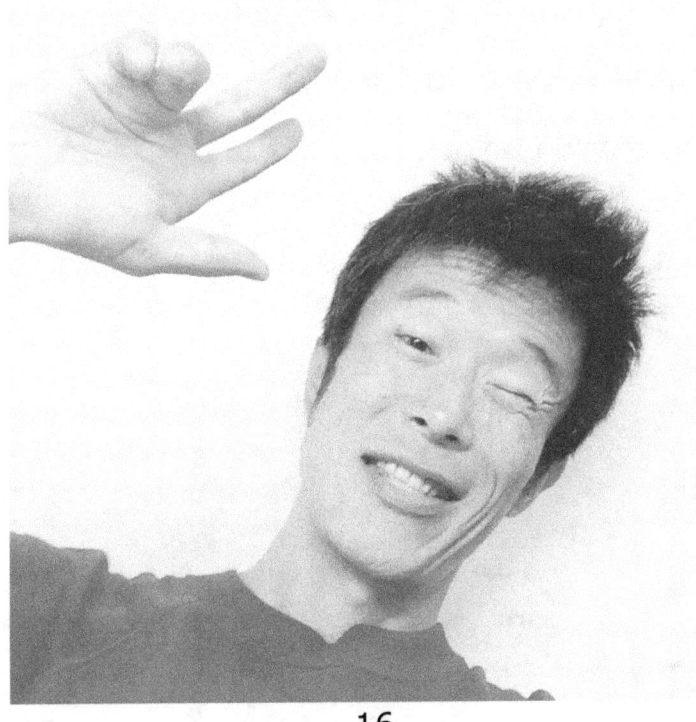

Chapter 5: 3 Rules of "Ninja Cure"

Set out basic rules, Tips to Health & Beauty.
1. Create an environment for success.
2. Cure/prevent colds.
3. "Reset-Relax" happens in just 8 seconds.

Description:

1. Create an environment

Cut or limit caffeine, alcohol & sugar.

2. Cure/prevent colds

Hot 7: First aid for colds and flu
Navel Salt: Natural salt relieves many symptoms

3. "Reset-Relax" happens in just 8 seconds.

Reset-Relax: At any place, any time
- For your good night's sleep and amazing performances.

Mantra: Activation of the brain

More information below:

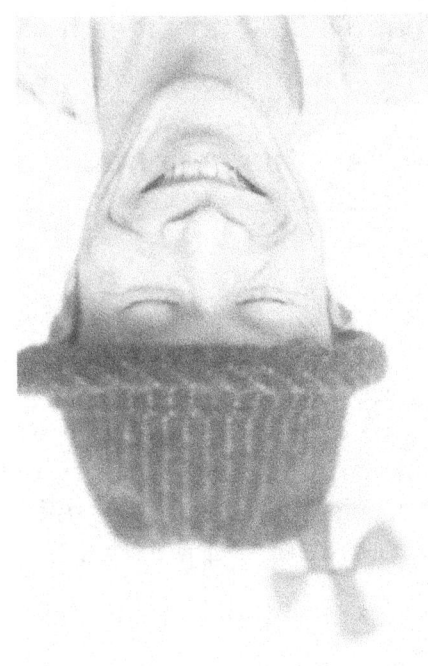

Chapter 6: Ninja Drink

Revolutionary fresh-squeezed vegetable juice recipe:

Makes 2 servings.

Ingredients:

1 medium carrot, cleaned
2 or 3 medium potatoes, cleaned and peeled
1 medium apple, cleaned and seeds removed from the white pith
Juice of 1/2 lemon, cleaned

* Get rid of the green-places of the potatoes.
* Take a potato with no buds.

Directions:

Process all ingredients, except lemon, in a juicer, not a blender. Squash the lemon to release the juice. Low-speed rotation is a better way as possible to get the nutrition alive. Of course, it's OK to squeeze them, wrapped in gauze, after grating the ingredients with a grater. The usage of pomace is up to you. I usually use them for supper. They do outstanding performance as a secret ingredient.

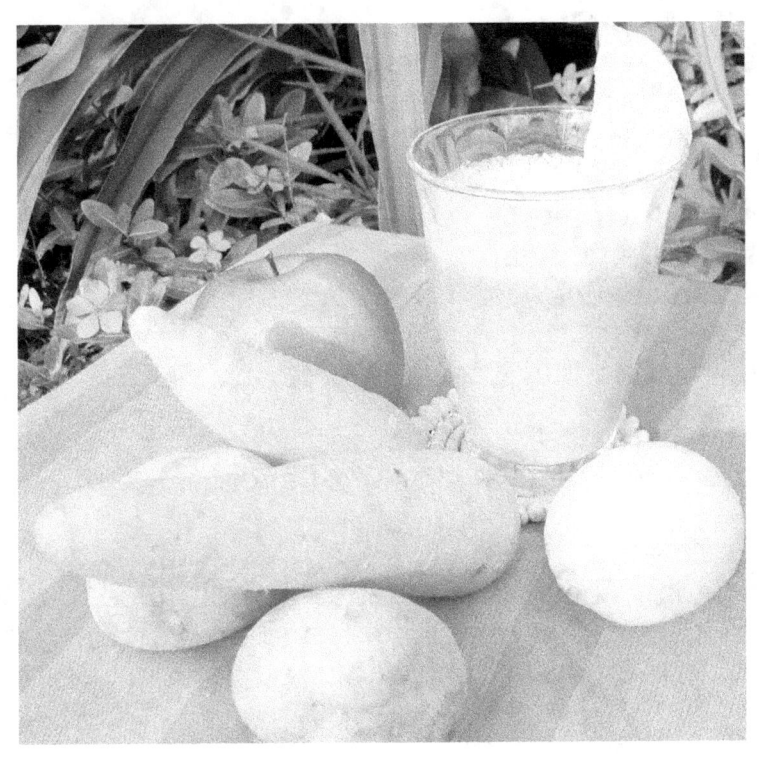

Chapter 7: Ninja Salad

Ninja Salad with Black/Golden Buddha Dressing, which is perfect for this boost/cleanse salad.

Black Buddha Dressing

Makes 2 servings.

Ingredients:
2 tbsp freshly squeezed lemon juice
2 tbsp fresh parsley leaves, chopped
1 clove garlic, minced
2 tbsp flaxseed oil, (or more if needed)
1 tsp black vinegar
1 tbsp white vinegar
1 tbsp soy sauce
Pinch sea salt
1 tbsp ground black sesame

Helpful hints:
* Frozen garlic turns into light flavor

Directions:
In a medium bowl, stir together lemon juice, flaxseed oil, salt, black/white vinegar and soy sauce gently. Combine the parsley and garlic. Adjust the seasoning.

Golden Buddha Dressing

Makes 2 servings.

Ingredients:

2 oz silken tofu (1/6 block)
2 tbsp freshly squeezed lemon juice
2 tbsp fresh parsley leaves, chopped
1 clove garlic, minced
2 tbsp flaxseed oil, (or more if needed)
1 tsp black vinegar
1 tbsp white vinegar
1 tsp soy sauce
2 tbsp yellow miso paste
Pinch sea salt
1 tbsp ground white sesame

Helpful hints:

* Frozen garlic turns into light flavor

Directions:

In a medium bowl, stir together the tofu, lemon juice, flaxseed oil, soy sauce, salt, black/white vinegar and miso paste gently. You don't want to mash them. Combine the parsley and garlic and gently mix in the tofu mixture. Adjust the seasoning.

Description:

Both dressings are selectively used. Basically, the black one for more warmth than the white one, because tofu has the function to cool. Mainly, eating the black one is advised. But each of them has all familiar daily ingredients. So, it's OK; you don't have to worry about that.

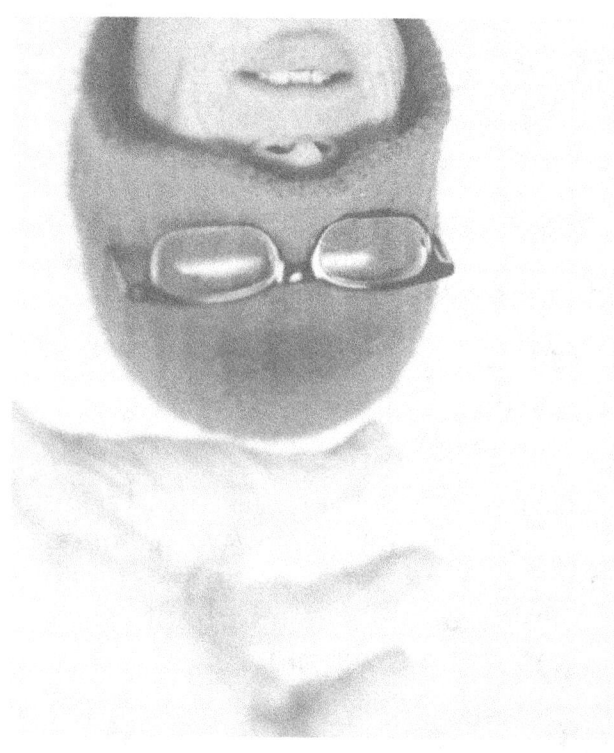

Ninja Salad

Makes 2 servings.

Ingredients:

1/3 medium carrot, cleaned
2 medium potatoes, cleaned and peeled
1/2 avocado, peeled, cut into 1/2-inch cubes
4 oz canned salmon
1/2 cup chopped scallions, green and white section
4 tbsp of grated, natural cheese

Helpful hints:

* Smoked salmon or raw salmon, as alternatives to canned salmon
* Soak the potatoes, peeled in water, for 2 minutes

Directions:

In a medium sized bowl, using the largest holes of a cheese grater, grate the potato and carrot (as you would cheese). A food processor with a grating blade will also work, but manual operation is the best. Add salmon and avocado. Pour the Black/Golden Buddha Dressing over the vegetable mixture. Sprinkle sliced scallions and grated cheese, and finally black/white sesame on the top. Serve with whole wheat bread or inside a pita.

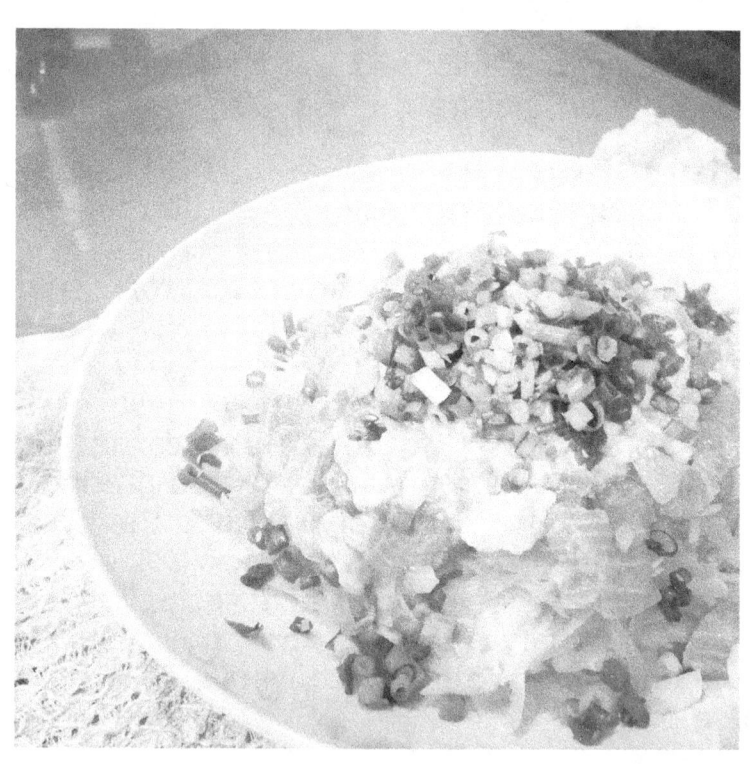

The primary effectiveness of *Ninja Salad/Drink:*
1. Antiphlogistic
2. Boosts your body & mood, builds up resistance to disease.
- Boosts your stamina, Prevents weakness, Prevention of illnesses.
3. Lets the blood flow well, gets the wastes out.
- Improvement of metabolism, Activation of cells.

Status of the use of *Ninja Salad/Drink*
1. Situations where you want to avoid medication, such as during pregnancy or having symptoms that are no cure by the drugs.
2. During/After Colds/Flu, Chronic disease, Being busy.
3. Helping the effects of your remedy and producing amazing performances.

[Medical Conditions]
Chronic Internal Disease (Liver Disease, Kidney Disease,etc), Neuralgia,
Arthritis, PMS, Tiredness(by stress,etc), Obesity, Insomnia, Rough Skin, Autonomic symptoms, Cerebral Anemia, Dizziness, Constipation, Irritation, Diabetes, High blood pressure, Gout, Rheumatism, Meniere's disease, Nausea, Varicose veins, Collagen-disease, Gastric polyps, Heartburn, Blurred vision, Stiff Shoulders, Backache, Breast cancer, Uterine cancer, Lung cancer, Decrease in stamina, immunity, etc.

Origin of "Ninja Drink/Salad

We call a carrot Ninjin and a potato Jagaimo in Japan. Nin of Ninjin and Ja of Jagaimo were added, and came out *Ninja*. As you may know, *Ninja* originally meant a Japanese soldier. They usually worked in the underground, like 007. They are guys of patience and loyalty. Now, if you're in any situation, I'd like you to dig up your passion. Ninja is like the path of a lightning bolt that you should count on. You're not alone. Here is a tip for success:

1. 「勇気」 Courage to try; nibble some at first
2. 「根気」 Patience to continue with some
3. 「意気」 Spirit to create your healthy life

Have a nice life :D

I genuinely hope that you will get strength like a *Ninja* when you come by genuine wellness with *Ninja Cure*.

Chapter 8: The Potato

Potato is known as a popular vegetable all over the world. No matter what the conditions, like hot or cold weather it is tough, it grows. The potato was brought to Europe by Columbus from Central America in ancient times. It's been told that the potato was one of the necessities for Napoleon continuing to advance. In France, "Pomme de Terre" stands for potato, but translates directly as "Apple of the earth". There is also a saying: "Taking a potato daily keeps a doctor away". Meanwhile, Philippinos even eat raw potatoes, called "Singkamas". You might have already eaten raw potato as salad.

Why is potato good for your health and beauty? Well, let's see two big reasons, below:

1. Treasure house of vitamins & minerals
2. Anti-inflammatory, Anti-stress, Adrenal cortical hormone-like

Rich in Vitamin C: Vitamin C of the potato is protected by starch, therefore it is hard to break, when it is cooked. Vitamin B1 is essential for the metabolism of carbohydrate, as a coenzyme. So, what is known about the role of vitamin C? You could say "skin". Vitamin C is a nutrient that is essential for the synthesis of collagen in the body. Collagen is made of proteins that are composed of amino acids. In brief, vitamin C is a common enzymatic cofactor used in the synthesis of collagen. Moreover, vitamin C does a lot of good things for the body. Vitamin C is a cofactor in at least eight enzymatic reactions.

I've been drinking *Ninja Drink* every day since October, 2009. Do you remember the beginning of this book? My history of weakness? Many of my symptoms have gradually improved. The first time I took it, I was really impressed with *Ninja Drink,* because I clearly felt that just some sips boosted me. Just like that, there was no doubt about adding it to my daily work- this really works for me, with confidence. Which of my symptoms is improved? Let me see: all chronic things: Anemia, Headache, Toothache, Autonomic nervous symptoms, Irritability, Dizziness, Fatigue, Neuralgia, etc. How about that? It seems like a miracle happened to me. But, all of this is true, fortunately.

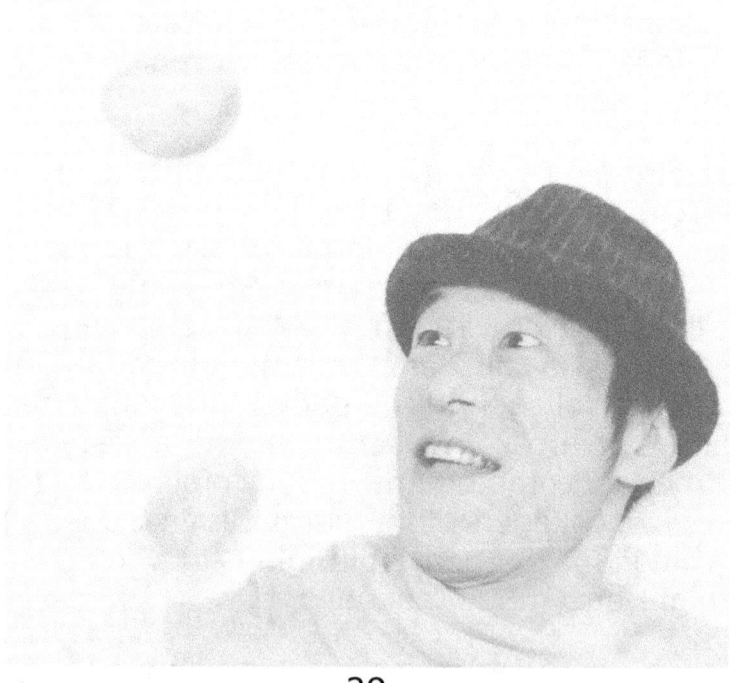

You know that knowledge of science and Oriental Medicine are saying that *Ninja* is genuine, safe and successful for us. Dr. Nabeshima, who told me the recipe of *Ninja Drink,* had been doing treatment activities in the United States for over 40 years. And he and *Ninja Drink* were very helpful for the grateful people around him. They have also helped my health. I just want to share those successful events with you. During my life, *Ninja Drink* has progressed to a revolutionary salad recipe. That is *Ninja Salad.* This was a totally awesome encounter. A puzzle has been completed beautifully. Tips I have met in my road of research have become one. I have continued eating *Ninja Salad* daily since December, 2013. *Ninja Drink* in the morning, *Ninja Salad* in the evening- that's one of my daily routines. One of the good reasons to have this salad is for chewing well, rather than drinking juice. Therefore, It's better to have *Ninja Drink,* with the action of your mouth like chewing, also. As previously stated, chewing promotes the secretion of saliva. I'd like to recommend to you 5 days per week at first.

And now, I have to tell you about my family, friends and patients that have gotten health with *Ninja Cure*. My wife was in trouble for health. She was also a department store of disease. History of her symptoms are Autonomic nervous symptoms, Alopecia, Asthma, PMS, Swelling, Rough skin, etc. When I met her, and she already had no hair at all. She had an inhaler and several drugs for her symptoms.

Well, she had gone and seen a lot of doctors, but no medicine cured her and no doctor told about any possible alternative remedies, such as food, Oriental Medicine, etc, that she should consider. Not at all. I am sure that there is an increasing number of doctors who don't prescribe only drugs. But, she hadn't got any successful opportunities for cure until she met yasuhirA iDee. Yes, that's me. At the beginning, we started a remedy of decreasing drugs, but gradually, because she had a weakness issue in her mind. It depends on the state of a person how long a period drugs should be kept away. So, I had to know how serious the symptoms were. More or less, chronic symptoms are often tough to improve. Especially for chronic symptoms, I say that there are no magical instant remedies- there's no shortcut. Doing the genuine routine daily is the only way to success. That's for sure. Ok, let's get back to my wife's story. As a result of this daily routine, she was able to lose weight healthfully. Healthy metabolism causes wholesome weight-loss, getting rid of your extra fat. Therefore, because of *Ninja Cure* and my treatment, she has gotten wellness. Of course, she is still human, and once in about 3 months, she has a headache or tiredness. But they are more milder than before. She has become able to easily get back to a wellness state when she's in some trouble. Her body hair has been growing day by day. Downy hair has also grown on her head.

And then, about her mother, she had had rheumatism for 3 years when we met. But her pain disappeared in 3 weeks after she started to take *Ninja Drink*. She has no longer needed any painkiller since then. That was in January, 2010. She is continuing to drink *Ninja Drink* with her husband every morning, and to have a healthy, happy life. Those successful stories are only the tip of the iceberg. To be honest with you, I am sure *Ninja Cure* will keep giving many people achievement of happiness, supported by wellness, from now on. Now, it's your turn.

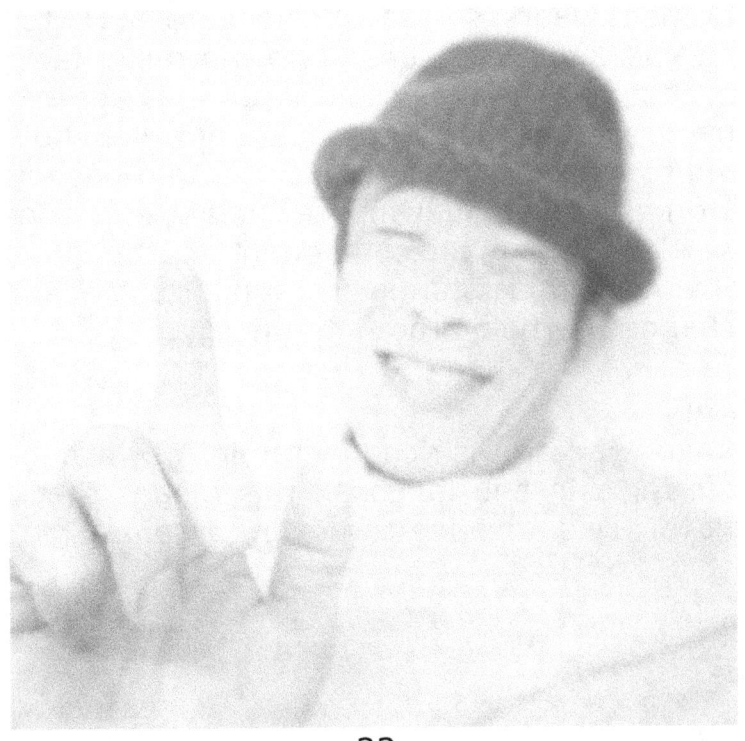

The additional story of the potato: This amazing vegetable, "potato", has wide-range cultivation and grows even in poor land. Have you ever heard of solanine as an alkaloid in potato. Solanine originally means "Sun", as the word is known as poison. But if you always throw away green tubers and sprouts that have toxic content, of course, they are OK to eat. I also wrote about this caution about solanine in my *Ninja Salad/Drink* recipe part. Moreover, the part of the potato to eat has a little bit of solanine, as well. But according to the researcher, a human body weight of 50 kg needs to eat 2.5 kg to become affected at once. There's no human who can eat a lot of potato at the same time, but I say, just in case, never do such a thing. Anyway, my wife and I have eaten them every day for many years, so I say it's going to be OK to have *Ninja Salad/Drink,* for sure. As a matter of fact, it is known that solanine has several powers: anti-cancer, anti-bacterial, anti-viral and anti-tumor. We should be grateful to avid researchers. Also, potato has vitamin B1, 3 times the amount in rice, and the calories are half of rice. The main component of the potato is carbohydrate, and vitamin B1 supports the enzyme that changes carbohydrate into energy.

Carrot:
As you know, carrot is rich in vitamin A, which plays a big role for skin and mucosal, this means they have benefit for eyes, arteries and every organ.

Of Course, your brain is one of the crucial parts that works by healthy blood circulation. So, memory ability could be improved by making the flow of blood better too. Well, it is said from old days that carrots make people lovable.

Oriental Medicine regards the autonomic nervous system as one organ. Its healthy function boosts your body and mood. The hypothalamus is the control center of the autonomic nervous system. The hypothalamus is located in your brain. According to Oriental Medicine, the kidney is related to the brain, spinal cord, reproductive system, etc. Moreover, the kidney has the function of warming the body from the inside, as the heart of all internal organs. We call the kidney "gin-腎", and now, you know that they are crucial organs and the vital systems to live, obviously. On the other hand, the potato is also good for your kidney and liver, and that means crucial organs in Oriental Medicine. This is it: *Ninja Salad/Drink* has great benefit for every organ and every cell and makes you smile and boosts your body and mood hilariously.

Remember: the flow of blood transports oxygen, nutrition and wastes in your body. As you know, the human body works successfully when the blood spreads evenly in every part of the whole body. The healthy blood cures one's body and mind, eventually. To sum up, healthy function of organs causes an original harmonious balance throughout the body. The state of good balance with each organ functioning properly is what the health is all about.

Please let me say something about potato again. From a natural point of view, potato has been used as one of the successful remedies: putting the potato paste on the area of arthritis and bruise and providing relief for inflammation of arthritis and gout. That's not only in Japan, but also worldwide. They are not useless at all, just because they are old. I want you to know there are lots of natural remedies which are explained scientifically today.

You can take *Ninja Salad/Drink* every day. As you know, they are not artificial drugs but natural vegetables. So there are no side effects. But the excrement may become a little bit softer for people who tend to sensitive intestine in the first week. However, you're gradually going to get used to it. So did I. You can drink it with confidence, from small children to elderly persons. The articles based on great experiences and success tell us the tips of health in "Shen Nong Ben Cao Jing-神農本草経". In Oriental Medicine, those ingredients belong to the most tender category. And now, you do not need to diet anymore, because *Ninja Cure* takes the extra fat off your body healthfully. Physiological function will have worked smoothly. We can call it *Ninja Diet*.

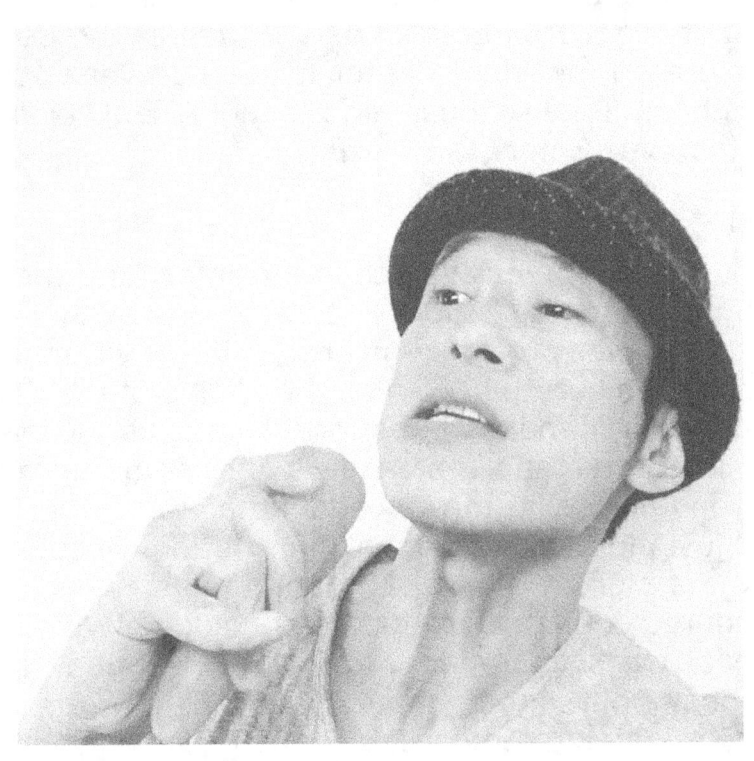

Garlic:

Another great reason of *Ninja Salad*:
A perfect package of vitamin C and dietary fiber, garlic brings a synergistic effect. It is the result of intense research by Dr. Motoki Yamanaka and Dr. Yoshisuke Enoki. Garlic promotes the keeping of water-soluble vitamins longer in the body, which means a fresh and young state continues longer. I genuinely believe that's great news not only for each and every person who hopes for wellness and beauty, but also for athletes, performers, and artists.

Apple:

As you know, apples are rich in enzymes, and there is the famous quote, "Apple keeps disease away". It is said that apples promote the absorption of vitamin C in the body. So potato known as the "Apple of the Earth" and apple itself makes the effort twice to us. No way; I think it's more than that. I always say this tip about food, and please let me say again that each ingredient is not just plural of nutritional information. Of course, I think it is a great thing that many things are going to be figured out by science/technology. Why not? Besides, we live among a lot of information- some might say right, some might say left. Finally, it's up to you. Still lemon is lemon. It's even not the only answer of 1 + 1. "Magic's just science that we don't understand yet," by Arthur C. Clarke. Today, in Oriental Medicine, scientific explanations have been developed in research organizations around the world. But there are still many parts of nature unexplained scientifically.

Sometimes, my patients say that it's like magic, when they got success. However, you may not prefer the noun "magic". In other words, they are facts. *Ninja Salad/Drink/Methods* and my treatments are all facts which mean genuine, safe and successful. The truth is always simple.

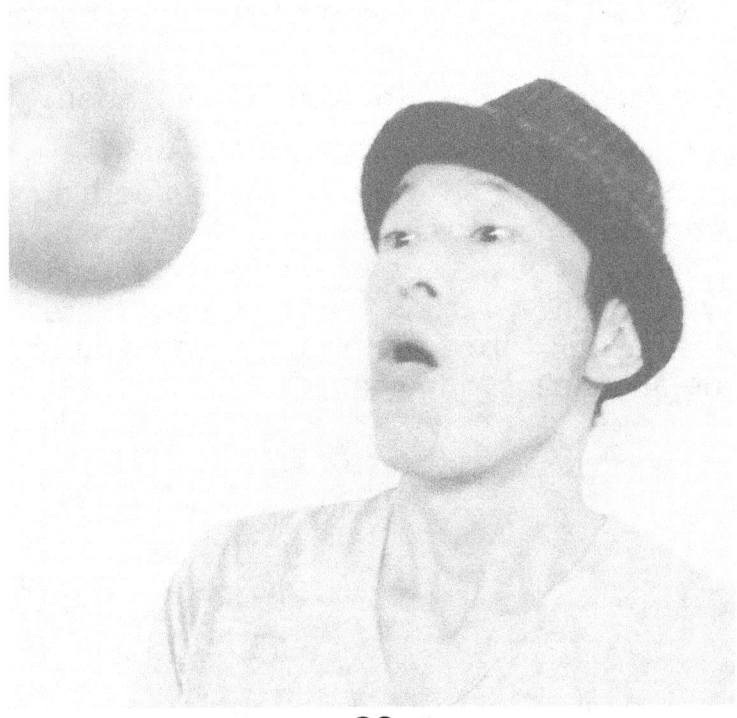

Chapter 9: The Bean

「食」 Eat naturally

「小豆」 "Adzuki Bean"

The primary 3 effects of "Adzuki Bean":

1. Improvement of swelling
2. Makes your body warm and boosts up resistance to disease
3. Cleans your kidney, which also means your liver, Cleanse: Diuretic, Constipation

「黒豆」 "Black Bean"

The primary 3 effects of "Black Bean":

1. Benefit for heart, kidney and liver
2. Makes your body warm and boosts up resistance to disease
3. Boosts and Cleanses: Diuretic, Constipation

Do you have a cuisine using beans in your hometown? Are the seasonings sweet, spicy, or something else? Well, there are some thoughts of Food-Cure in Japan which say that beans are great for your health and beauty. Especially, Adzuki/Black beans are great. For instance, adzuki provides primary improvement for swelling and cleans kidneys.

The meanings of internal organs in Oriental Medicine
「腎」 = "GIN" = Kidney
The 3 primary meanings of "GIN":
1. Brain, Spinal cord, Ear, Throat, etc.
2. Reproductive system
3. Native spirit from your parents

According to Oriental Medicine, the kidney is related to the brain, spinal cord, reproductive system, etc. So, kidney means the spirit itself from your parents. The kidney has the function to warm the body from inward, as the heart of all internal organs. Certainly, the kidney is a very crucial organ in your body. And we call the kidney "gin-腎".

Low-fat, high protein is a good quality. What is the popular menu cuisine of beans in your country? Or what do you say "cuisine" in your place? I hope that there is a Japanese food shop in your town. However, you should eat vegetables, not only meat, obviously. You know that you can't keep going by eating only meat. That's not a good idea for your health and beauty. Of course, the protein is necessary nourishment for your life. I recommend an adzuki bean, more or less soybean, as well, because, adzuki is low-fat and high protein in a good quality. The popular way to eat it is boiling.

Japanese food has many boiled and seasoned dishes, and the seasonings of them tend to be sweet. For example, Oshiruko, Zenzai, Boiled pumpkin and adzuki bean. Mix adzuki with chocolate, cookies, or cake as a dessert, etc.

Makes 2 servings.
Ingredients:
80 g Black or Adzuki bean
800 ml water
2 inch dashi kombu (dried kelp) or seaweed, roughly
chopped
2 tsp bonito flakes (Dried fish, sliced thinly)
1 medium dried shiitake (mushroom), roughly chopped
1 tsp soy sauce
pinch sea salt

* If you don't have dashi kombu or bonito flakes, you
can use seafood stock. Bonito flakes and dried shiitake
can be omitted. Meanwhile, seaweed that you can get
still works for the stock, instead of dash kombu. When
you can get only raw shiitake, dry them in the sun for
several days, because sunshine boosts the nutrition of
ingredients.

Directions:
Place the beans in a medium pot and cover completely
with water (approximately 800 ml). Add in the dashi
kombu (or seaweed) and dried shiitake. Soak for one
hour. After that, bring the broth up to a boil and then
add in the salt and give it all a stir, gently. Reduce heat
and cook for about 20 minutes. During cooking, add
the water for the amount reduced. Add in the soy
sauce and put a lid on it for a minute. Taste and season
with salt and soy sauce as needed.

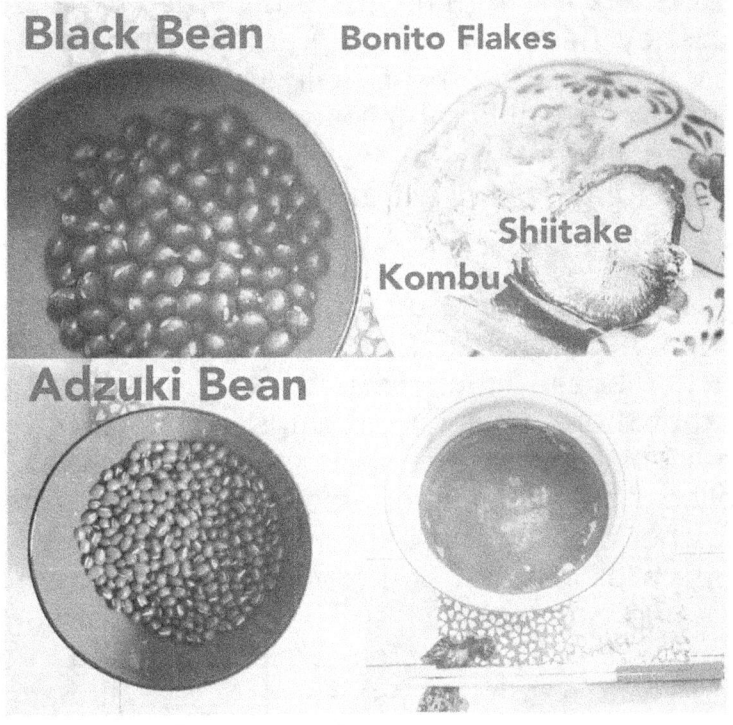

Black Bean   Bonito Flakes

Shiitake

Kombu

Adzuki Bean

Descriptions:

This recipe is my way daily, and no need to remove any ingredients, because I want you to eat all of them. In accordance with medical textbooks, Dietary fiber: Excretion; suppresses absorption of extra salt; suppresses pylori, that is the cause of gastric cancer; gastric ulcers, and induction of apoptosis in cancer cells. It is rich in vitamins, minerals and omega-3 fatty acids. They have a flavor ingredient, "Umami", that causes the secretion of saliva. And the surface whiteness of dashi kombu is sweet, so it's OK that you just clean it gently with water. Just as in Japanese cuisine, eating it plain, without spice, is recommended. I hope you like it.

Eat a seasonal food naturally, and season it minimally for your healthy life. The menu is possible from products made in Japan with your original. Of course, I think that there are a lot of things in accord with your cuisine. There are the canned, boiled beans in Japan, as well. But, I think it's not a good idea for your health. Watch the label on the backside, by all means, when you buy a processed food. You should avoid artificial sweeteners and additive stuff. What kind of sugar is popular in your country for sweet seasoning? People are led to three directions: sweetness, saltiness and greasiness by the modern huge food industry. The movie "Food, inc" said that, too. To be honest with you, they are already in the ingredients- a seasonal food already has all seasoning.

Remember: Eat seasonal foods naturally; season them minimally for your healthy life. By the way, do you cook usually? If you do not, please try it and have fun. Good luck:)

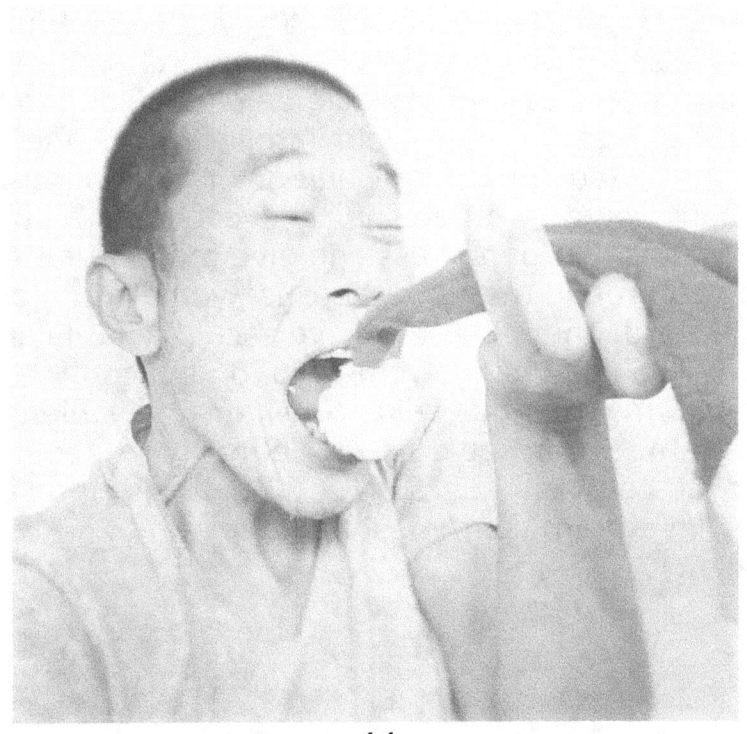

Chapter 10: The Smilefie

We know that science/technology has been developing day by day, and of course that's great; but too many people today are living with issues such as disease, depression, conflict, etc. and that gap is tough to close. Remember: we have a natural healing power originally, an amazing doctor works throughout our body, and it's a great idea to count on "Family Doctor" as much as possible. Moreover, there are many things you can do for your achievements in the future. One tip- why don't you go with a smile :) As you may know, a happy hormone is released and explains why smiling is good for your health and beauty.

As a matter of fact, "It takes only 17 muscles to smile. It takes 43 muscles to frown." Why not smile? Just by taking a selfie photo with your beautiful smile when you start every day; or it would be a good idea to take a picture of each other- your family, friend and your neighbor. And next, uploading on Instagram or Facebook, or any other sns. You can play a role in increasing smile/happiness and give the gift of lifelong health all around the word, because you are one of the whole world. Therefore, I believe each of your hilarious actions could change the world peacefully. For example, my hilarious selfie *Smilfie* is available in my Instagram. So, if you'd like to learn more about this idea, you can visit:
http://instagram.com/yasuhira_idee
Thanks :)

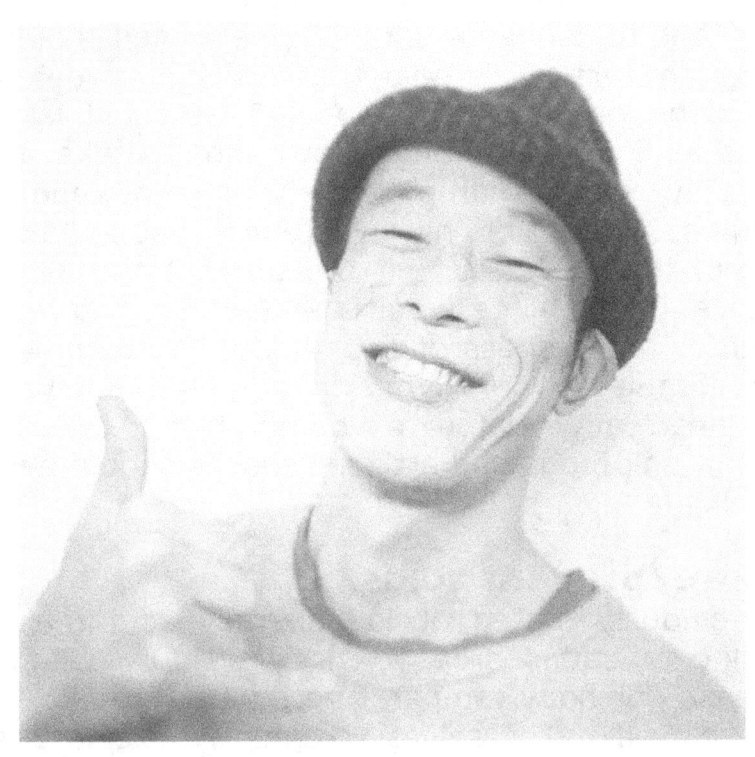

Chapter 11: The Create

3 Rules of "Ninja Cure":
Set out basic rules, Tips to Health & Beauty.

1. Create an environment for success.
Cut or limit caffeine, alcohol & sugar.
I want you to know that ingredients made from hot areas tend to cool your body. Those stimuli should be used with care. It is said that artificial sweeteners hinder the production of blood. That could lead to coldness and overeating. You should take care, especially with children, elderly persons and any weakness. That's not only sweeteners, but could be all artificial things, because it is said that the artificial chemical things hinder your flow of blood, and tend to promote the coldness of your body. In other words, they stimulate your sympathetic nervous system. They are really related to your body and mood. Of course, junk foods and artificial snacks should be cut, as well.

2. Cure/prevent colds.
As previously stated, it is generally said that our immune functions drop down by 30-40% when we decrease our body temperature by 1 degree. We can balance well by ourselves, originally. The issues of balance and temperature cause most chronic diseases and many troubles of your physical status and mind. As you know, the human body works successfully when the blood spreads evenly in every area of the whole body.

The activation of cells requires oxygen, moderate nutrition and temperature. What brings those things? Yes, your blood is all about. There are a lot of research and procedures about fever in Western Medicine. But you may know that there is less research about methods for coldness. That is to say, most people would know the ways that they should cool down when one has a high fever. Meanwhile, have you ever heard any method for boosting your body? Yes, we have. Please refer to the following.

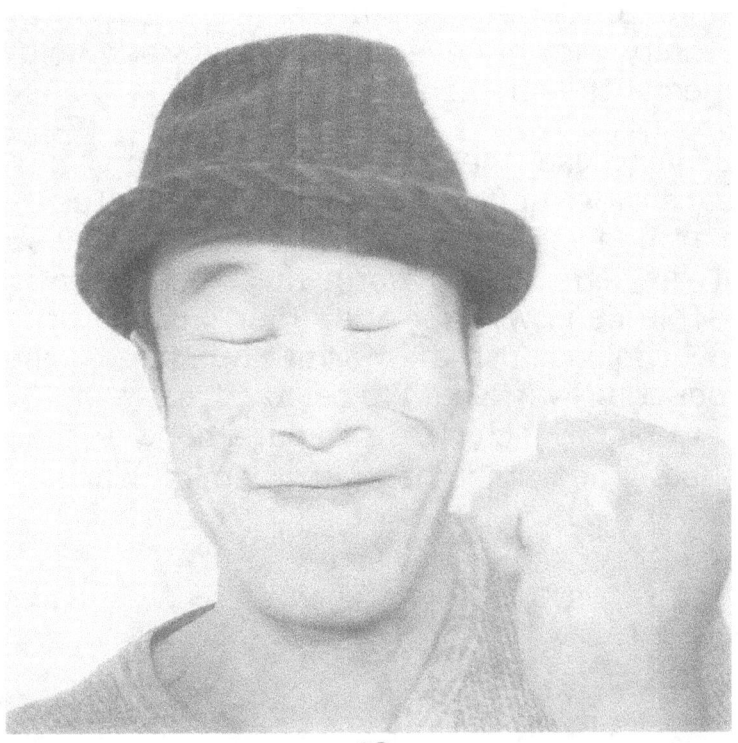

"First aid for colds and flu"

Natural Self-Care
「大椎大温」 "HOT C7"

「手当」 in Japan
Easy & tender remedy
Initial symptoms of cold: If you felt a chill on your back, what would you do? Do you have any method of your own? You may know that there are many natural remedies all around the world. In this situation, just beneath the nape of the neck is the very good key area that is very effective to get rid of cold. There is one of the acupuncture points called "GV14- 大椎". I'll introduce you to a very easy and quick Self-Care that I recommend. It's very helpful Self-Care, and I have an opportunity with my everyday patients and volunteer activities at the stricken area, too.

We usually use the warmth of burning moxa to approach the acupuncture point. But when there is no moxa around you, what should you do? Don't worry. It is still very effective to warm the crucial area with a disposable hand warmer and dryer, instead of moxa. Moreover, please use the warmth of a hand if there is no product for warming. We call the treatment "Teate-手当" in Japan, which means to put a hand on the place of trouble. The human hand itself emits heat.

They are really helpful, not only as daily remedies, but also an aid for the state of being stricken. When I volunteered in the stricken area to support with the treatment, I brought a disposable hand warmer. They have really worked. So, I am happy that you share and expand this helpful remedy ,HOT C7, to people concerned with the place who needs any support. Of course, let them be known to someone important to you, like your family or friends as one of the daily Self-Cares. Thank you:)

The primary effectiveness of "HOT C7":
1. Initial symptoms of colds/flu
2. Coldness

Status of use "HOT C7":
1. Situations in which you want to avoid medication, such as pregnancy, and people who have symptoms that have no cure by drugs.
2. Helping with the effect of your remedy

Ingredients:
Disposable hand warmer or
Ginger Oil, Hot Balm, etc.

Directions:
Put a disposable hand warmer on your area beneath the nape of the neck. Please see the figure below. That's it. Simple, isn't it?

This is a safe, tender and genuine method that has been supported by many years of experience. This is Natural Self-Care, so it's very tenderly useful for a pregnant woman who cannot take medicine, and is also for elderly persons and children.

「寒邪」 "Cold-Wicked"

A cold begins with your area beneath the nape of the neck. It is said from ancient times that the Cold-Wicked comes in from that area. Cold-Wicked is called "Kanja-寒邪" in Oriental Medicine. The cold syndrome is the boss of 1,000 diseases. A chill often leads to all kinds of diseases. When you feel a chill on your back from the neck, please try this Self-Care *HOT C7*, and then, take some cozy-up drink and sleep warmly. That's a very tender method to drive out a cold early. In addition, when you have no disposable hand warmer, you can use the warmth of dryers, electric heater, Ginger Oil or Hot Balm on the area-*HOT C7*. This is a natural, tender, safe and totally genuine method that was supported for many years of experience. No side effects. But, when you use the products to warm, please be careful about a burn. Please do not put the hand warmer on skin directly. By all means, please try some and take care. Thank you:)

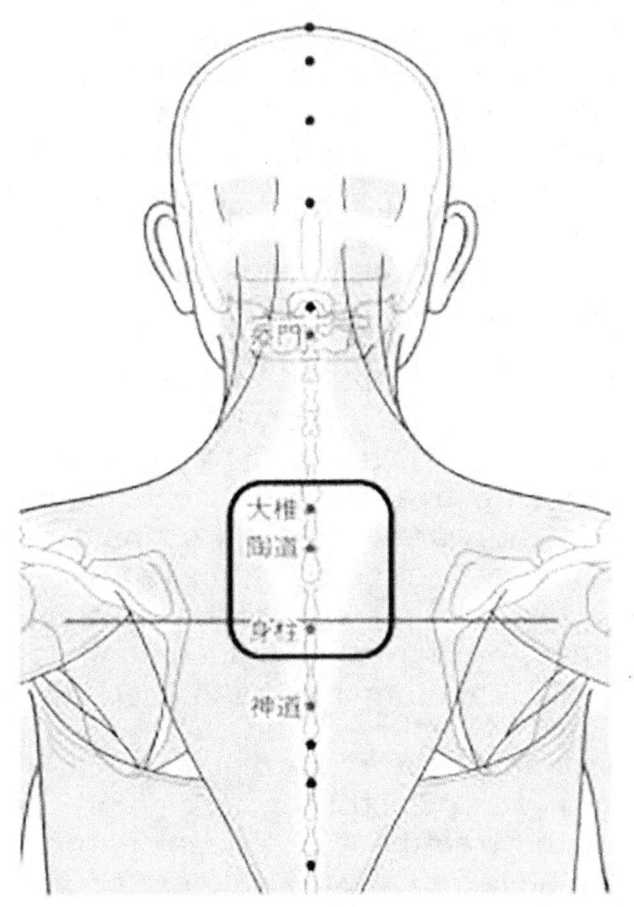

"Natural salt relieves"

Natural Self-Care
「臍塩」"Navel Salt"

「手当」in Japan
Easy, tender remedy
Do you know that the navel is a very good key point that has an influence on the whole body? That is one of the acupuncture points called "Shinketsu-神闕". I will introduce you to a very easy and quick Self-Care that I recommend. It's very helpful Self-Care opportunity for my everyday patients and in my volunteer activities at the stricken area, too.

We usually use the warmth of burning moxa on the salt and acupuncture point. But when there is no moxa around you, what would you do? Don't worry. It is still very much effective to warm the navel with a disposable hand warmer and dryer, instead of moxa. Moreover, please use the warmth of a hand, if there is no product for warming. We call the treatment "Teate-手当" in Japan, which means to put a hand on the place of the trouble. The human hand in itself emits heat.

Natural salt helps the state of the stricken. When I volunteered at the stricken (tsunami) area with support of the treatment, I brought natural salt and tape. They have really worked. Yes, all you need is natural salt and tape.

So, I am happy to share and expand this helpful remedy, *Navel Salt,* to people concerned in a place that needs any support. Of course, let them be known to someone important to you, like your family and friends, as one of the daily Self-Cares. Thank you:)

The primary effectiveness of "Navel Salt":
1. Pain Relief
2. Makes your body warm, builds up resistance to disease
3. Relaxation

Status of use "Navel Salt":
1. Situations in which you want to avoid medication, such as pregnancy, and people who have symptoms for which there is no cure by the use of drugs.
2. Helping with the effect of your own remedy

[Medical Conditions]
Abdominal pain, Vomiting, Diarrhea, Coldness,
- Menstrual Pain
- Infectious diseases, such as the Norovirus and Colds
Constipation,
Sleeplessness,
- Irritation, trouble of the autonomic nervous system, Backache, and totally as relaxation.

Ingredients:
Natural salt (Except refined salt)
Adhesive-bandages (about 70mm×30mm)
Disposable hand warmer

Directions:
Put salt on your navel, literally. The amount of the salt is about 1 tsp. Put an adhesive-bandages on it, so that it won't spill. That's it. Simple, isn't it? It's a safe, tender and genuine method that is supported by many years of experience. This is natural Self-Care, so it's very tenderly useful for pregnant woman who cannot take medicine, and is also for elderly persons and children. Natural salt has a lot of minerals and warmth itself. It has been said from ancient times that the salt protects you from a wicked thing or event, other than as the seasoning. The use-by date is about 1/2 day.

When there is any symptom of an infectious disease and you are tired more than usual, put a disposable hand warmer on the *Navel Salt*. In addition, you can give warmth of your hands to the *Navel Salt* and use the warmth of the dryers, as well. But, when you use the hand warmer and dryer, please be careful about a burn. Please do not put the hand warmer on skin directly.

My teacher, Kenshi Nabeshima experienced the atomic-bomb in Nagasaki, Japan during his school days. He and his friends cured vomiting and the diarrhea that were a symptom of being atomic-bombed and survived by *Navel Salt* and moxa treatment.

Moreover, my pregnant friend got over the symptoms of vomiting and the diarrhea of the norovirus, in a night. She had cured their symptoms by the next morning by the *Navel Salt* using a disposable hand warmer, instead of moxa warmth. By the way, do you have natural salt? Please try some and take care. Good luck:)

* Illustrator: Hagi Warae

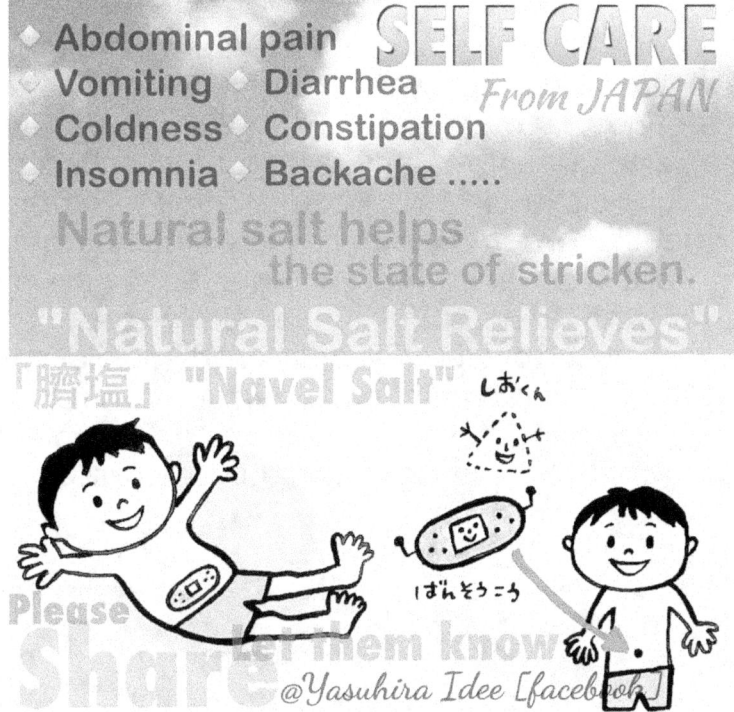

3. "Reset-Relax" happens in just 8 seconds.

"At any place, any time":
For your good night's sleep and amazing performances.

Natural Self-Care
「押優安眠」 "Reset-Relax"

In life, there are some crucial moments. You should prepare for your success. What do you think about your conditioning in order to lead a daily effort for achievements. I hope everything is all right, without any trouble. But, unfortunately, there might be a case that does not work well. And now, I believe that amazing performances require a well-balanced state of health.

Daily routine is very important for your health. Do you have any method of your routine, such as food, exercise and yoga? Does it work? Well, you could say good-bye to sleepless nights when you become a master of relaxation. You could show off fabulous performances when you become a master of daily reset. More than anything, in order to simply spend your life with a beautiful smile. So please, let me introduce you to very simple and quick natural Self-Care that I recommend. Even if your routine is working, use it to become even better. If you don't have any method, please make this the first step, by all means.

The keywords are..."Reset-Relax". You can do this at any place, any time. Why do you need to get some relaxation under pressure? You know that people can't spend all day in full throttle. That's a function of the sympathetic nervous system. For example, please regard the sympathetic nervous system, as switch-on. On the other hand, the parasympathetic nervous system is switch-off. Switch-off means relaxation. This is called the autonomic nervous system as the functions of the two. Most of the issues of sleeplessness are related to the strain of the sympathetic nervous system, which means the condition of not relaxing easily. Let's see the possible states. It is said that the biggest cause is stress that could not be let out on a daily basis.

[Possible states]
* Mental side
Sleeplessness
Constipation, Diarrhea,
Fatigue, Upset etc.
* Physical side
Trouble of the throat,
Stiff-shoulder, Backache etc.

It is said that the troubles of the autonomic nervous system mostly cause those symptoms. This means it could go well and you could be more easily cured when sick by becoming a master of relaxation and balance and by continuing natural Self-Care. Remember: "Health/Beauty is an art, won by 99%-SelfCare and 1%-genuine treatment." You might take the drugs when in trouble, but they should be avoided as much as possible. Please try to use natural stuff, because it is said that most of the artificial chemical stuff hinders your flow of blood and tends to promote the coldness of your body. They stimulate the sympathetic nervous system in the long run.

How stress beats you when under pressure:
[Mechanism]
1. Autonomic nervous system covers the capillaries throughout our body.
2. Stimulation by artificial stuff influences the sympathetic nerves system.
3. Sympathetic nervous system is stimulated, causing a shrinkage of the capillaries.
4. Blood circulation of your entire body is suppressed by shrunken capillaries.
5. Suppression of the blood circulation throughout the body leads to coldness.

Remember: The cold syndrome is the boss of 1,000 diseases. A chill often leads to all kinds of diseases. Cold-Wicked is called "Kanja- 寒 邪 " in Oriental Medicine.

「寒邪」 "Cold-Wicked"

Let's review this tip, the human body works successfully when the blood spreads evenly in every part of the whole body. For instance, throat, sensory organs like the ear and eye, of course the brain, heart, hypothalamus, etc. The hypothalamus is a playmaker of the autonomic nervous system that plays a crucial role in our functions of the natural side- literally, every organ you have. Moreover, they are all made of the cells. Activation of cells requires oxygen and moderate nutrition. What brings the nutrients and oxygen? That's right, your blood. The human body tends to get cold and chill from the waist and tips of your toes, as you know. Remember that cold day in winter. You might have felt your toes and fingertips very cold. It's just like that.

Why not massage the fingers and toes?
The fingertip is very connected to the brain anatomy and physiology by nerves. There is also an acupuncture point important for Oriental Medicine, which means it is related to organs. A tip: warming the hands and feet invites sleep because relaxation by the parasympathetic nervous system is activated. So wearing gloves and socks is one of the ideas to warm yourself for nice and relaxed sleep.

How to get some relaxation and reset when under pressure:

"Self-Massage"

Activities by hand can be said to be like a Shiatsu, rather than to be kneading dough. Shiatsu is used as finger pressure. That's the method for acupuncture point, as well. Push down on the skin surface.

Where?

Finger (Hand, Foot)
Crucial point is "two corners of the base of the nail-plate".
- Not Fingertip side, Lunula side
- Proximal nail fold area

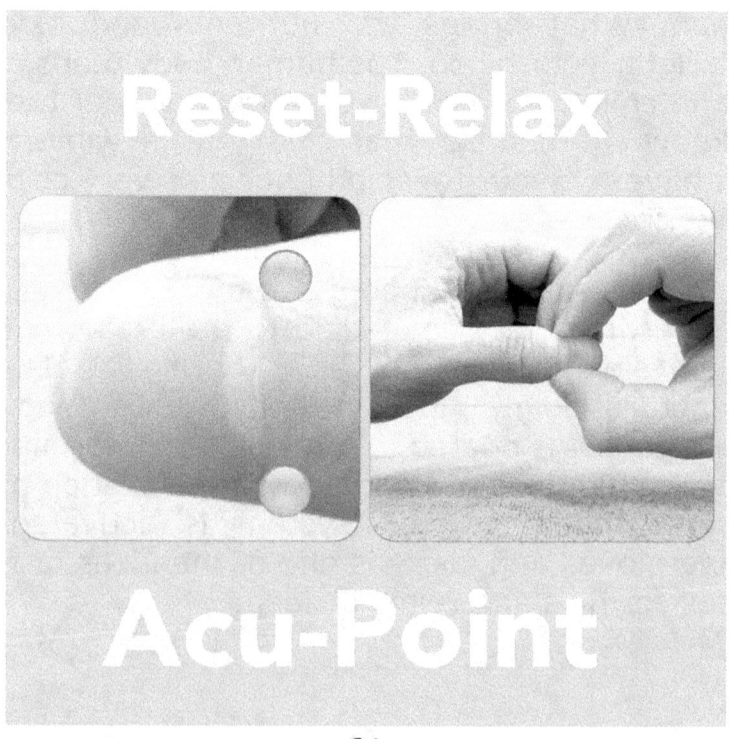

61

How?

Push those points with your thumb and index finger of your other hand, that looks like an OK-sign. The strength is about between comfortable and painful. Let's call that feeling "Comfo-Pain". Pick up the nail-tips slightly to get an appropriate stimulus the same as "Comfo-Pain". At the same time let's go massage up from the palm and the other side, the right and left side of your fingers and toes. Of course the palm of your hands and the arch of your foot, as well.

How long?

About 8 sec per one finger tip. It's a simple way, so it's very useful back stage before a performance, as well, not only conditioning daily.

How often?

You can do it whenever you need: when you're sleepy but you can't; want to sleep but you can't; freaking out in a nervous moment before a performance; etc. Natural healing power is activated because this remedy influences the autonomic nervous system gently.

It is a safe, tender and genuine method that has been supported by many years of experience. This is natural Self-Care, so it's very tenderly useful for a pregnant woman who cannot take medicine, and is also for elderly persons and children. Please try natural Self-Care for your amazing performance and daily health:) I hope you like it.

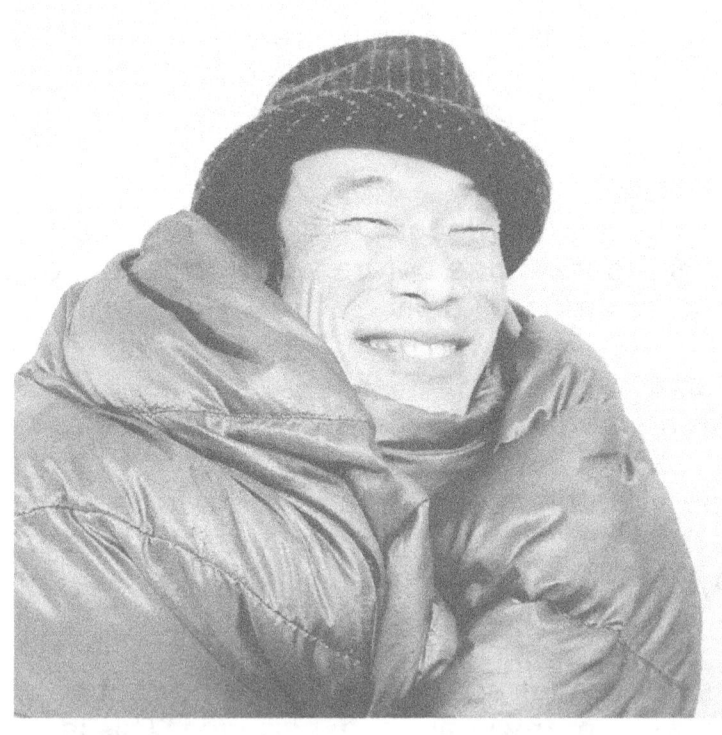

"Activation of the brain"
For your good night's sleep and amazing performances.

Natural Self-Care
「振柔脳活」 "Mantra"

Do Mantra every morning/night. Have you ever done a mantra? Mantra is known as a method of yoga. I have been doing yoga since 2000. Now, let me introduce to you a very simple and quick Natural Self-Care that I recommend. Some arrangement is added to it, that I learned. Mantra is a harmony of initiation and termination. The vibration of mantra brings us a clue of health. Generally, people use a word "O-M". But, I'd like you to say it like this. Well, I suggest 2 more words as mantra.

"O-M"
"A-Un" "あうん" in Japanese
"Amen" in English

Next, the second half of the word should be vibrated longer than the vowels before. Close your lips and say/vibrate "M, Un, n".

M of "O-M"
Un of "A-Un"
n of "Amen"

Be aware of the area to your brain from the temple when you say/vibrate the second half of the word. Have you ever had the experience of voice training? Resonance of the nasal cavity is going to be a tip to learn. Remember that Oriental Medicine regards the autonomic nervous system as one of the organs. Scientifically, it affects organs such as the heart, respiratory and digestion. So, its healthy function boosts your body and mood. The hypothalamus is the control center of the autonomic nerve system. Do you know where the hypothalamus is? Yes, it is in your brain. In other words, this remedy is a massage by vibration of your mantra. And now, you're going to be able to massage the brain yourself. What a wonderful Self-Care!

Finally, I think it's a good idea that you pick your word as the mantra. But, please notice the place of the vowel when you choose the word. So, what's the mantra at your place? I hope you like it. Good luck:)

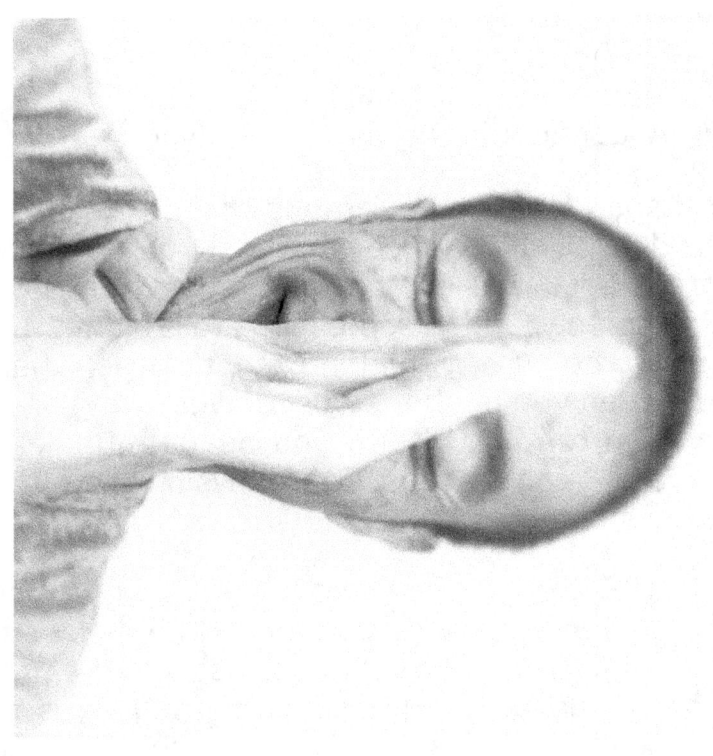

66

Chapter 12: Ninja Method

5 tips for your healthy life.

The Ninja Method inspires your life.

食, N, Natural Food + Eat naturally, with a smile
想, I, Idea + Smile causes the hormones to go around your body nicely
動, N, Natural Movement + Smile
笑, J, Joy/Smile + Laughing
息, A, Abdominal Breathing + Laughing

This method comes from famous thoughts that were organized by Ekiken Kaibara, who wrote "Yojokun". That great book was written in the Edo era, 1600s. *Ninja Method* has added some ideas to it by me. It has 5 pillars as the way of thinking. That's a very helpful method, when you might get lost on your way, or want to transform to more health and beauty. Thinking of Health-Care, I can say this idea shows a wide range of foundations and uses.

The key is "Smile"- that will make you happy, for sure. There's no health and beauty without a smile. Happiness loves wellness. As you may know, a happy hormone is released, explaining why smiling is good for your health and beauty. Your face helps you show the world how you are. As previously stated, "It takes 43 muscles to frown. But it takes only 17 muscles to smile!" That's from another great book, "An Illustrated Adventure in Human Anatomy".

Moreover, the state of frowning stiffens your body and mood. Why don't you use your power for something in a positive way? How does that sound?

Smile relates to all tips in a good way.

食, N, Natural Food + Eat naturally, with a smile. Cook with a smile. You can also sing a song along the way.

想, I, Idea + Smile causes the hormones to go around your body nicely. A smile promotes the regular function of the hormones. It's very important to have smily, positive thoughts for your health and beauty.

動, N, Natural Movement + A smile is a good exercise itself, and laughing is an even better way that uses your abdominal breathing.

笑, J, Joy/Smile + Laughing

息, A, Abdominal Breathing + Laughing Let's move your belly by Laughing!

「腹式呼吸」 Abdominal Breathing
Abdominal breathing is friendly, the simplest routine exercise, and is also the most important motion. Also, you can approach the autonomic nervous system with it. The hypothalamus is the control center of the autonomic nerve system. The hypothalamus is located in your brain. In Oriental Medicine, the spirit of "gin-腎気" lives in the hypogastric area and is very related to the brain. In other words, the brain is connected to the hypogastric area. That's the reason that you should train the hypogastric area by abdominal breathing.

「息」Breathing

Breathe to be relaxed when you're in trouble. Be aware of breathing out more than breathing in. Let's start- 1-breathing in, and 2-breathing out. Breath-in like a sponge in water. When you let a sponge go from your hand in water, the sponge absorbs water naturally, so just like that.

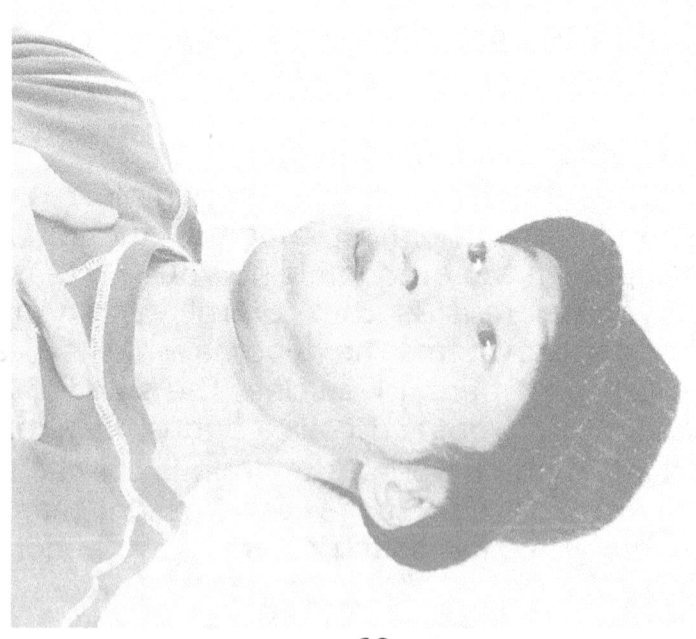

More tips for your healthy life.

「生旺墓」 "Sei, Oh, Bo"
Metabolism =
Born 「生」 , Flourish 「旺」 , Grave 「墓」
Nothing lasts forever- a fact that is common to all living things. But it's up to your idea whether your life flourishes with your true colors shining through, even if you can't fight fate. The grave is a destination forgiven only by a completely ready person. "Sei, Oh, Bo"- that means the metabolism itself. At the point of both views, physically and mentally, metabolism is the key.

"Smile for no reason. 'Cause the sun shines for no reason." Why not smile?

"An unrestful remedy is no remedy at all."

"Haste stands against you, Gentle steps stand by you."
Life is not a sprint-race, but like a marathon, not a postseason, but like a regular season in major league baseball. You can't spend the days at full throttle. In daily remedy, you should always do natural things first.

"The biggest stress is a soul."
Life is like taking a walk with your soul. And now, don't forget smiling a lot along the way."

「汗」 *Sweat your rust out.*
「吐」 *Breathe them out.*
「下」 *Detoxify them down.*
「和」 *Neutralization.*
「汗吐下和」 *"Kan, To, Ge, Wa"*
That's what metabolism is all about.

"I can't go a day without being excited ;)"

"The pleasure that you have gotten so far can't steady the excitement to follow."

3 control systems which are important to human health are...
   1. *Immune*
   2. *Hormone*
   3. *Autonomic nervous*
Working these systems in a good balance lets your life become healthy and beautiful.

"You could be someone leaned on, while you learn Self-Care."

"Health/Beauty is an art, won by 99%-SelfCare and 1%-genuine treatment."

"There is no mistake, except in no longer doing your own routine."

"Down the road with a smile, Health will find you."

These 3 things that are connected to nature cannot be long forgotten: Eat, Breath, Q.
1. 「食」 *Eat naturally*
2. 「息」 *Breathing*
3. 「灸」 *Q = 灸 (kyu) = Moxa*

「丹田」「腎」「原気」
"Hypogastric, maṇipūra-cakra"
Also, the place that conceives a child. That is to say that the hypogastric is important in breathing. The whole world says that the hypogastric is a crucial place.

「自然治癒力」
"Vis Medicatrix Naturae"
"Spontaneous Healing"
"Natural Healing Power"
Heal naturally. Let it alone to do that. Entire human's body tends to be balanced in a good way naturally. That's what Spontaneous-Healing is all about. A medical treatment and self-care is just a little help at the right time and in the right place. Remember:) Health/Beauty is an art, won by 99%-SelfCare and 1%-genuine treatment.

"Are you a Wild One?"
Wildness and Knowledge help you out of any kind of trouble. Both of them bring you the clues that help you figure out something, like dreams, success and wellness. Remember: Wildness and Knowledge when you are stuck.

"Knowledge & Digging"
Knowledge is a bridge for dreams. You can reach higher, if you dig wherever you like, deeper.

"Hey diseases, if you'll excuse me, I'd like to get back on Dream Train."

"Your soul is naturally coming from someplace positive."

"Grateful = Faith to all,
Faith = Pray to all"

"Necessities for world peace":
Passion, Knowledge, Wellness,
Wellness loves Smiles :) Nothing Beats Smiles!

「夢 」 *Dreaming*
"Never give up on your dream! Anything can happen."

Thanks, Good luck :)

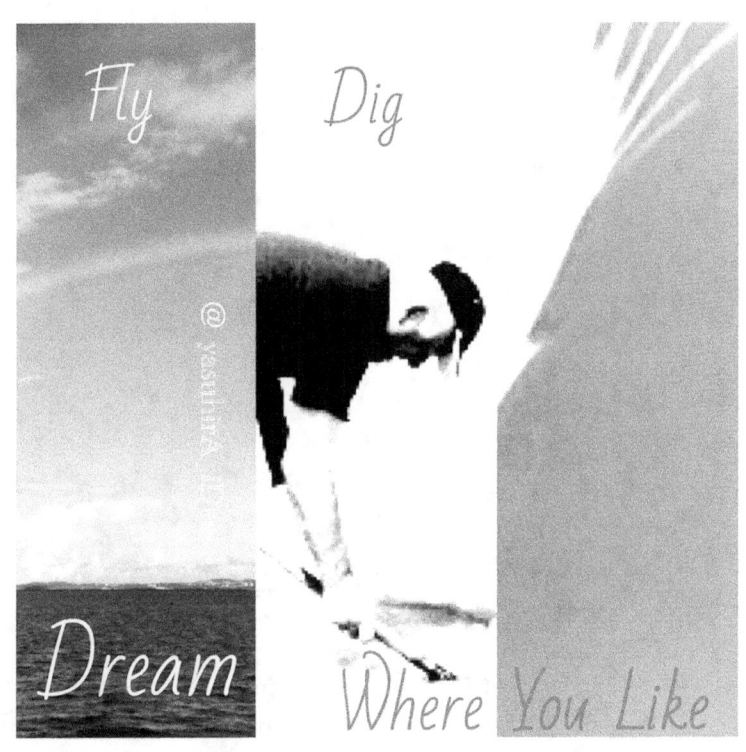

Fly　　　　Dig

@
yasuharA_ill

Dream

Where You Like

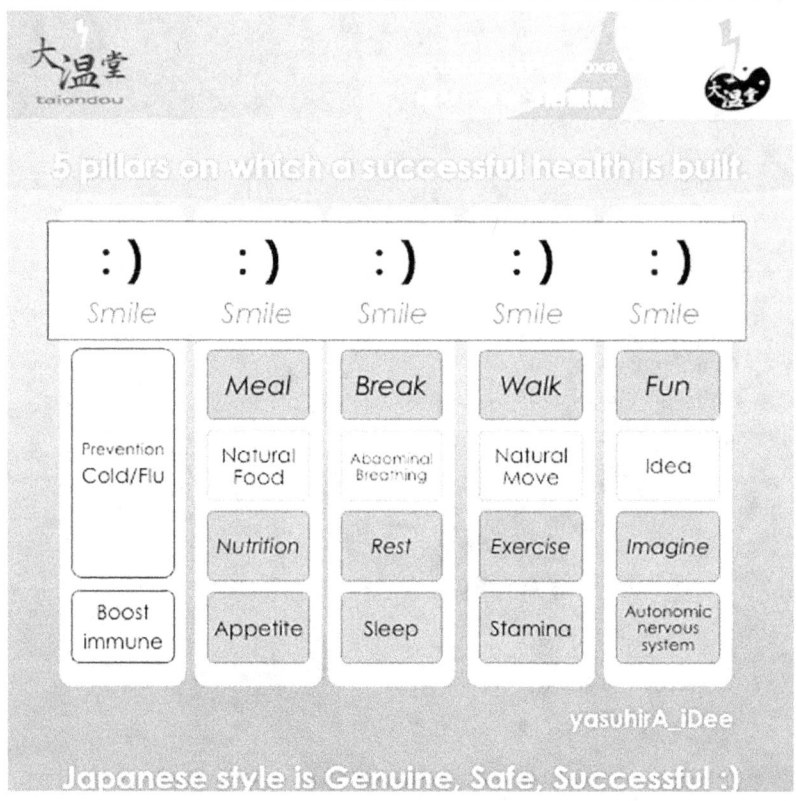

5 tips for your healthy life:

The Ninja Method inspires your life.
食, N, Natural Food + Eat naturally, with a smile
想, I, Idea + Smile causes the hormones to go around your body nicely
動, N, Natural Movement + Smile
笑, J, Joy/Smile + Laughing
息, A, Abdominal Breathing + Laughing

Notes

Please note: This book is only intended to provide general information and is not specific medical advice. You should consult with your own healthcare professional before altering or beginning any course of treatment. yasuhirA iDee is not responsible for any losses, damages, or claims that may result from your decisions and you are strongly encouraged to do your own research prior to any decisions you make.

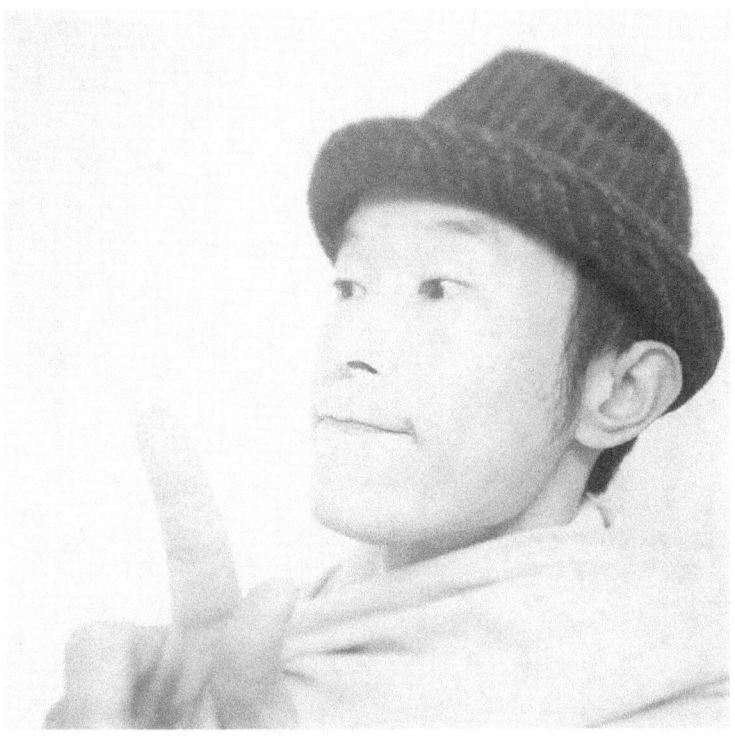

References

"The Ningen Igauk" since 1938

"Shizenryoho"
by Yuriko Tojyo

"An Illustrated Adventure in Human Anatomy"
by Kate Sweeney

"Keiraku Keiketu"
by IDO NO NIPPON SHA

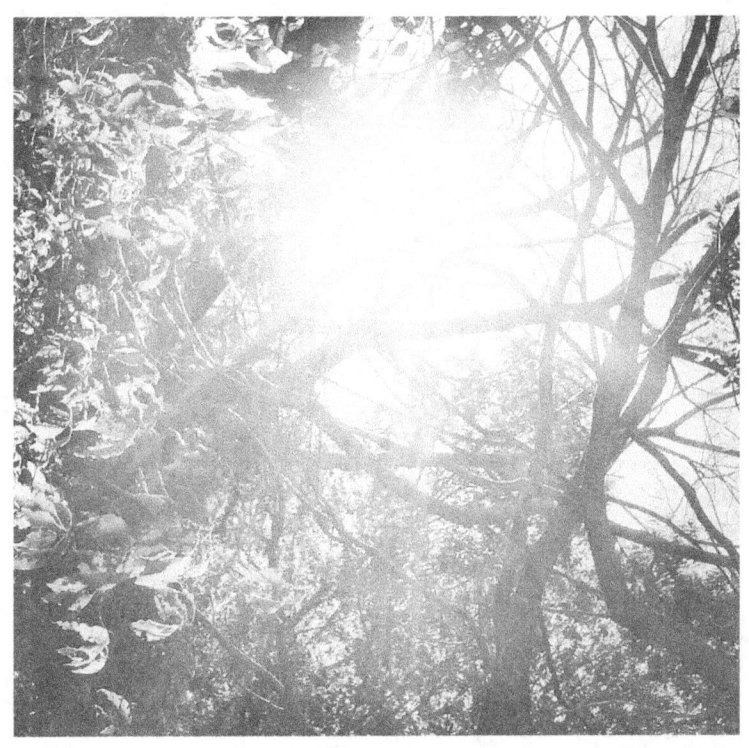

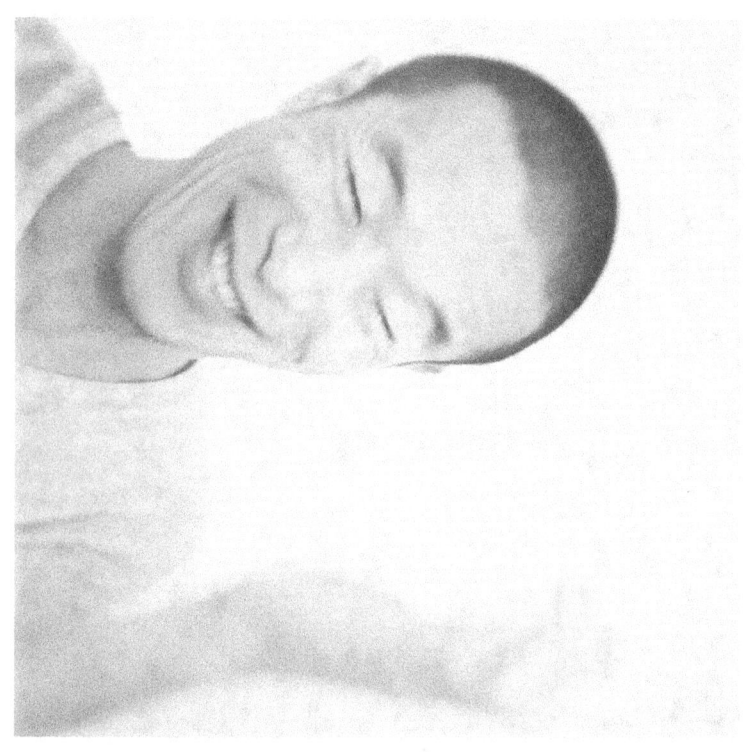

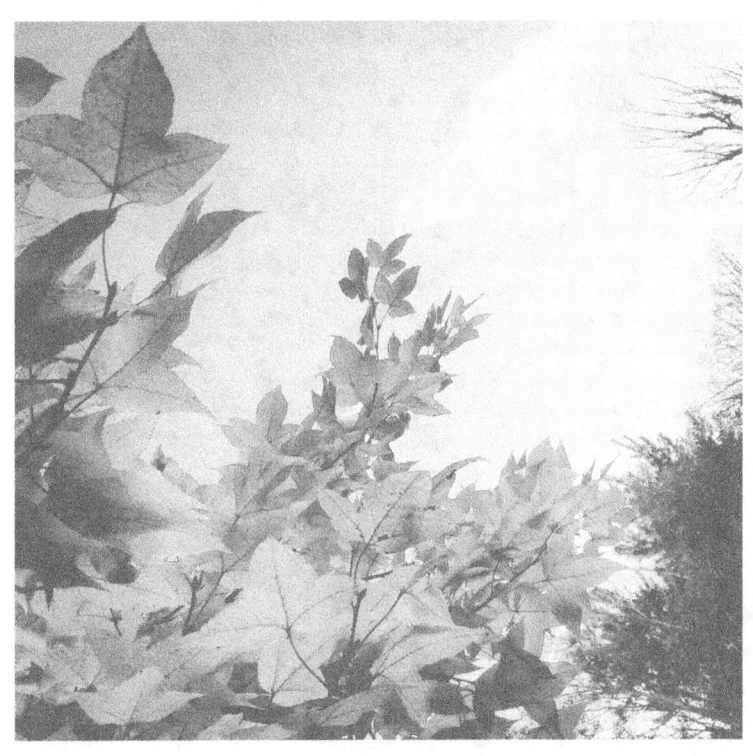

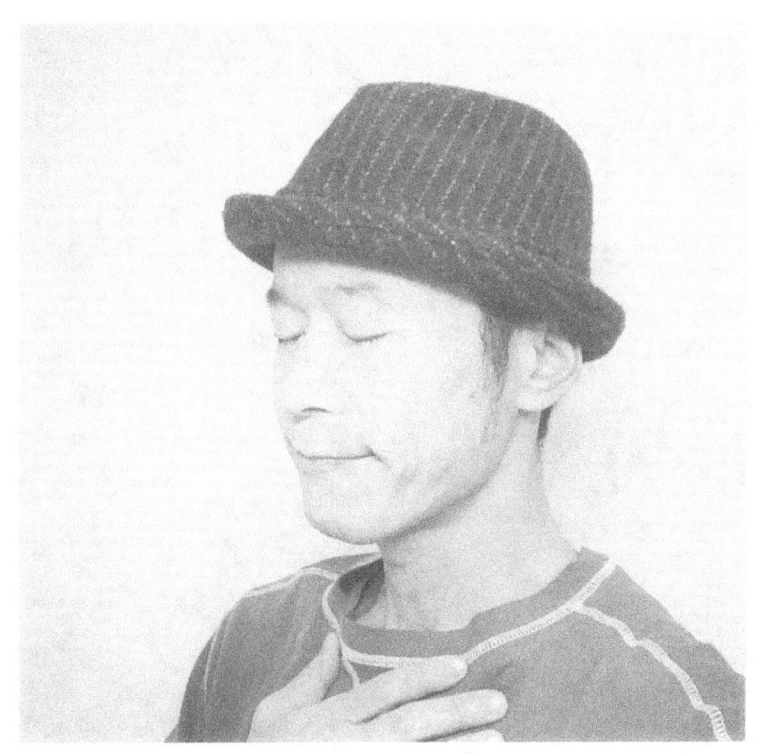